Rahma Gargouri
Rym Khemakhem
Nesrine Kallel

Radiological aspects of medisatino-pulmonary sarcoidosis

Rahma Gargouri
Rym Khemakhem
Nesrine Kallel

Radiological aspects of medisatino-pulmonary sarcoidosis

ScienciaScripts

Imprint

Any brand names and product names mentioned in this book are subject to trademark, brand or patent protection and are trademarks or registered trademarks of their respective holders. The use of brand names, product names, common names, trade names, product descriptions etc. even without a particular marking in this work is in no way to be construed to mean that such names may be regarded as unrestricted in respect of trademark and brand protection legislation and could thus be used by anyone.

Cover image: www.ingimage.com

This book is a translation from the original published under ISBN 978-620-6-70746-2.

Publisher:
Sciencia Scripts
is a trademark of
Dodo Books Indian Ocean Ltd. and OmniScriptum S.R.L publishing group

120 High Road, East Finchley, London, N2 9ED, United Kingdom
Str. Armeneasca 28/1, office 1, Chisinau MD-2012, Republic of Moldova, Europe
Printed at: see last page
ISBN: 978-620-7-95368-4

Contents

CHAPTER 1

A) <u>INTRODUCTION</u>:

Sarcoidosis is a disease of unknown cause that mainly develops in patients aged between 25 and 45 (1,2).

The clinical presentation of sarcoidosis depends on the intensity and duration of the inflammation and the organs involved. Mediastino-pulmonary involvement is the most common. The phenotypes of the disease are highly variable, ranging from completely asymptomatic forms with pulmonary alterations found incidentally on routine chest X-rays to sub-acute and acute clinical pictures with dilapidating and sometimes atypical pulmonary lesions posing a diagnostic dilemma (3). Clinical, biological, radiological and pathological evidence is often required. Histological evidence is provided by the presence of an epitheliogigantocellular granuloma without caseous necrosis, while excluding other causes of granulomatosis, essentially tuberculosis (4,5). In the majority of cases, therapeutic management must take into account the initial spontaneous evolution of the disease. Therapeutic intervention depends on the organs affected and the severity of the disease. Corticosteroid therapy is the first-line treatment and is therefore not always indicated. In symptomatic mediastino-pulmonary forms, the thoracic CT scan will play a pivotal role in assessing the evolution of the disease.

treatment.

CHAPTER 2

B) <u>PATIENTS AND METHODS</u>

TYPE OF STUDY

This is a retrospective descriptive and analytical study covering a period of twenty years, from January 2002 to December 2022, in the Pneumology Department of the Hédi Chaker Hospital in Sfax.

TARGET POPULATION

The study included 35 confirmed cases of mediastino-pulmonary sarcoidosis. The diagnosis was based on a suggestive clinical, radiological and biological presentation, the demonstration of epithelioid and gigantocellular granulomas without caseous necrosis, and the exclusion of any other granulomatous disease (4,5,6).

In this study, the diagnosis of mediastino-pulmonary sarcoidosis was based on the diagnostic approach illustrated in Figure 1 :

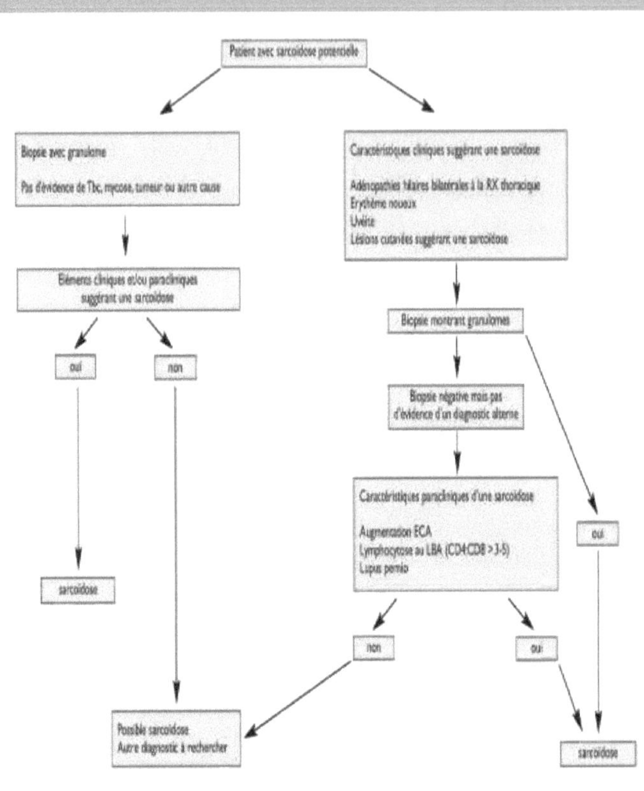

Figure 1: Approach to a patient suspected of having sarcoidosis (after

Swiss Medical Journal, 2005; Sarcoidosis: new concepts
pathogenic and therapeutic approaches to an 'old' disease) (7).

The following table shows the diagnostic elements used in our work to diagnose mediastinopulmonary sarcoidosis:

Table I: Clinical, radiological,
biological and histological elements used in the diagnosis of
mediastino-pulmonary sarcoidosis.

Evidence suggesting mediastinopulmonary sarcoidosis	Features

Clinic	Combination of intra-thoracic involvement with : 1. Skin disorders (erythema nodosum, lupus pernio) 2. Neurological damage (damage to the VII cranial nerve) 3. Ophthalmological damage (uveitis) 4. Syndromic association (Heerfoldt syndrome)
Radiological	1. Bilateral hilar adenopathies (the most suggestive radiological feature).
	2. Diffuse micronodules predominantly in the upper lung regions on standard chest X-ray. 3. Peripheral lymphatic micronodules on chest CT.
Organic	1. CD4 / CD8 ratio > 3.5 (the most specific biological element) 2. Moderate lymphocytosis in BAL fluid 3. Abnormally high ACE levels 4. Disturbed phosphocalcium balance 5. Tuberculin test (for BK)
Histological	Granuloma tuberculosa without necrosis caseous (identification of this histological aspect in the lymph nodes hilar and mediastinal lymphatics is of great diagnostic value)

METHODOLOGY

Data were collected from patients' medical records using a pre-established form to meet the objectives of the study. The following data were collected:

3.1.Socio-demographic data

3.2.Lifestyle habits

3.4.Clinical data on sarcoidosis

3.4.1. General functional signs

Fever, asthenia, anorexia and weight loss.

3.4.2. Thoracic functional signs

Dyspnoea, cough, chest pain, palpitations and haemoptysis

The severity of dyspnoea was subjectively classified according to

The Medical Research Council (mMRC) modified dyspnoea scale in five stages

(8) (Appendix 1)

3.5.1. Data from standard chest X-ray

The disease was classified into 4 radiological types according to the Siltzbach

classification (9): (Appendix 2)

3.6. Chest CT scan data

3.6.1 Data on lung parenchymal involvement

Elementary parenchymal lesions

- Micronodules

- Nodules

- Parenchymal condensations

- "Hyperdense areas of ground glass

- Crazy paving" appearance

- Peribronchovascular thickening

- Thickening of the septal lines

- Thickening of non septal lines

- Fibrosis lesions: Traction bronchiectasis,

Scissural distortion, bronchovascular distortion, intra-lobular reticulations, honeycomb images, fibrosis mass.

- Cavities

- Paracicatricial emphysema

- Aspergilloma

- Signs of pulmonary hypertension

3.6.2 Characteristics of typical lung disease :

- Typical parenchymal involvement in sarcoidosis consists of diffuse, bilateral, symmetrical elementary parenchymal lesions with a peri lymphatic distribution, predominantly in the upper and middle regions of the lungs (10).

- Typical fibrosis lesions are traction bronchiectasis, distortion and reticulation (10).

3.6.3 Characteristics of atypical lung disease

- Unilateral parenchymal disease

- Basal predominance of elementary lesions

- Atypical nodules: nodules with ground-glass halo, pseudotumour nodules

- Images in Basal honeycomb

- Atelectasis and bronchial stenosis

- Cavity lesions

- Post-obstructive bronchiectasis

- Military

- Pleural involvement: pleural effusion, pneumothorax

3.6.4 Distribution of parenchymal lesions in the lobes

Frequency of parenchymal involvement in each lobe

3.6.5 Predominance of parenchymal lesions

- Frequency of each predominant parenchymal lesion

- Predominant parenchymal lesion topography: Diffuse, upper and/or middle region, lower region.

3.6.6 Data on lymph node involvement

Adenopathy measurements were missing from the majority of CT reports, so this parameter was not studied.

Location of mediastinal lymph node chains

- Hilaires

- Paratracheal

- Aorto-pulmonary window

- Bifurcation group

- Under carenaries

- Anterior mediastinal

- Posterior mediastinal

Frequency of atypical lymph node involvement

a- Atypical location of adenopathies :

- Adenopathies of the posterior mediastinal chain

- Adenopathy of the internal mammary chain

- a- Diaphragmatic or cardiophrenic adenopathies b- Unilateral hilar

adenopathies c- Calcified lymph nodes

d- Necrotic adenopathy

Associated scannographic lesions

Dilatation of the trunk of the pulmonary artery, dilatation of the right cavities

and mycetomas.

3.6.7. CT classification of mediastinopulmonary sarcoidosis

C) <u>INCOME STATEMENT</u>

1. Prevalence

During the study period, 35 cases of patients with mediastino-pulmonary

sarcoidosis were recorded, corresponding to 0.13% of all hospitalisations in the

pneumology department during that period.

2. Clinical study

The functional signs of the patients are summarised in Table II.

Table II: Summary table of functional signs presented by

patients at the time of diagnosis.

	Number of cases	Percentage
General signs		
Fever	2	5.7
Asthenia	19	54.3

Anorexia	10	28.6
Weight loss	16	45.7
Thoracic signs		
Cough	28	80
Dyspnoea	29	82.9
0 mMRC	6	17
1 mMRC	19	54
2 mMRC	3	9
3 mMRC	3	9
4 mMRC	4	11
Chest pain	11	31.4
Palpitations	5	14.3
Haemoptysis	4	11.4

3. Radiological study

3.1 Standard chest X-ray

Chest X-rays were performed in the entire population.

study.

According to Siltzbach's classification, the radiological types most frequently encountered were type III in N=12 patients, i.e. 34.3%, and type II in N=10 patients, i.e. 28.6% of cases. (Figures 2, 3, 4, 5 and 6).

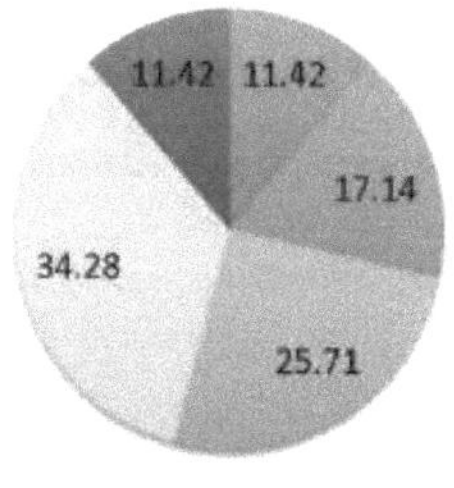

Figure 2: Radiological stages of the study population according to the Siltzbach classification.

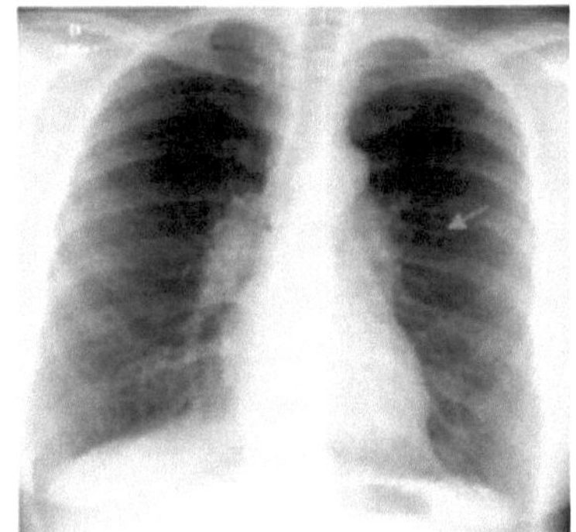

Figure 3: Front thoracic X-ray of a patient being followed for

stage I mediastino-pulmonary sarcoidosis.

Bilateral (   ), symmetrical, non-compressive hilar adenomegalia   .

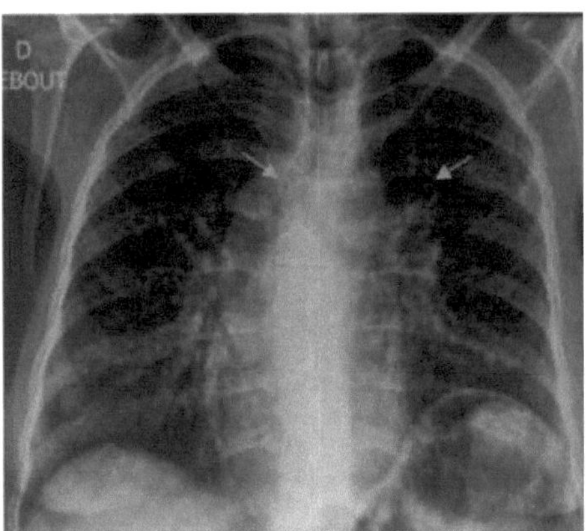

Figure 4: Front thoracic X-ray of a patient being followed for

stage II mediastino-pulmonary sarcoidosis.

Bilateral parenchymal involvement with bilateral hilar adenomegalia (   ).

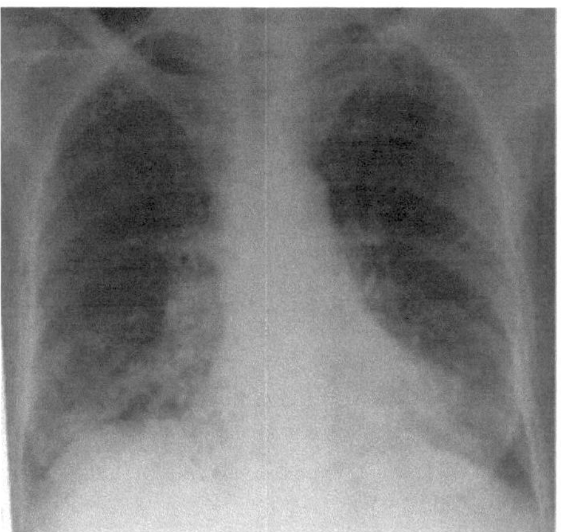

Figure 5: Front thoracic X-ray of a patient being followed for

stage III mediastino-pulmonary sarcoidosis.

Lung parenchymal infiltrates without associated adenomegaly

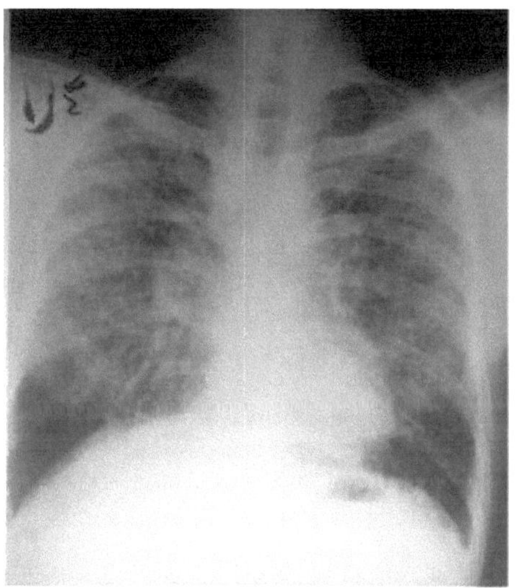

Figure 6: Front thoracic X-ray of a patient with stage IV mediastino-

pulmonary sarcoidosis.

Bilateral parenchymal involvement at the fibrosis stage.

3.2 Chest CT data

Chest CT scans were performed in the entire study population on discovery of the disease. The abnormalities found were sometimes multiple in the same patient, and were dominated by parenchymal involvement with elementary lesions present in 32 patients, i.e. 91.4% of cases. Lymph node involvement occurred in 30 patients (85.7% of cases), as shown in Figure 10.

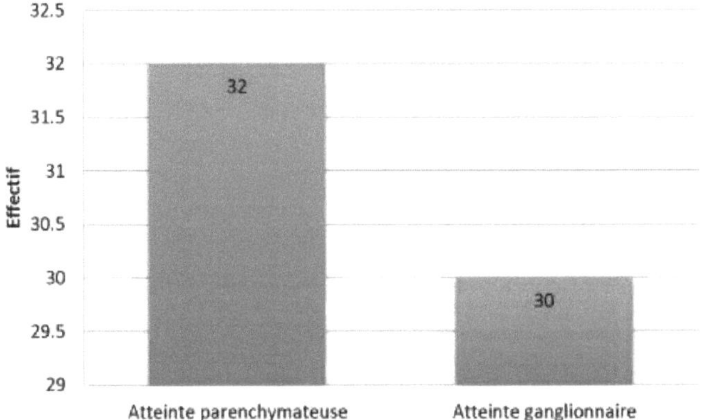

Figure 7: Distribution of the types of anomalies found on CT scan in

the study population.

3.2.1 Parenchymal disease

3.2.1.1 Characteristics of elementary parenchymal lesions

In our series, 32 patients (91.4%) had elementary parenchymal lesions, which are summarised in Table VII.

The most frequent parenchymal lesions were micronodules of perilymphatic distribution, bilateral, with clear and confluent contours found in N= 25 patients, i.e. 71.4% of cases. (Figure 8).

The subpleural and juxta-scissural location of the micronodules was highly suggestive of their perilymphatic distribution, sometimes giving a pearly appearance to the scissure, clearly visible on sagittal reconstructions (Figure 8).

In addition to micronodules, pulmonary nodules were noted in

N=18 patients, i.e. 51.4% of cases. In most cases, the nodules were solid, sub-centimetric in size and regular in outline. In some cases, the pulmonary nodule was surrounded by a collar of micronodules giving a characteristic "Galaxy Sign" appearance. (Figure 9)

Peri-bronchovascular thickening was found in 40% of cases in the form of a sleeve which engages the bronchial and vascular structures without any sign of compression or invasion. (Figure 10)

Septal lines were observed in N=12 patients in 34.3% of cases, and non septal lines in 20% of cases. (Figure 11).

Lesions suggestive of fibrosis were present in 7 patients, i.e. 20% of cases, such as traction bronchiectasis in 20% of cases, scissural and bronchovascular distortions in 20% of cases, and intralobular reticulations in 14.3% of cases. In contrast, fibrosis nodules and honeycomb were present in only 8.6% of cases. (Figure 12)

Cavitary lesions were present in only one patient. No cases of aspergilloma were noted.

Table III: Distribution of elementary parenchymal lesions in the study population.

Elementary lesions	Number of cases	Percentage
Micronodules	25	71.4
Nodules	18	51.4
Condensations parenchymal	7	20
Frosted glass	10	28.6
Crazy paving	2	5.7
Thickening bronchovascular	14	40
Septal lines	12	34.3
Non-septal lines	7	20
Fibrosing lesions	7	20
Bronchiectasis of traction	7	20
	7	20
Scissural distortion	7	20
Distortion bronch-		

vascular	5	14.3
Cross-links intra-lobular	3	8.6
Honeycomb	3	8.6
Fibrosis mass		
Cavities	1	2.9
Emphysema paracicatricial	1	2.9
Aspergilloma	0	0
Signs of PAH	3	8,6

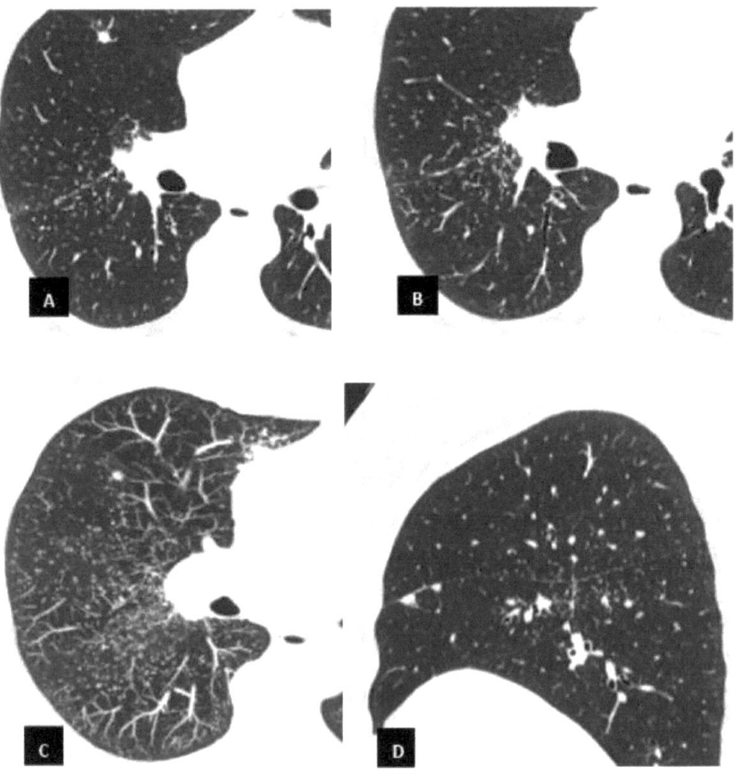

Figure 8: Micronodules of purely lymphatic distribution in a female 60-year-old woman with mediastino-pulmonary sarcoidosis, of

Micronodules with clear contours and sustained density in the centre and periphery of the secondary lung lobule in axial section (A, B), better highlighted in MIP mode (C). Sagittal reconstruction (D) confirms the presence of multiple juxta-scissural nodules, confirming the perilymphatic distribution of the micronodules.

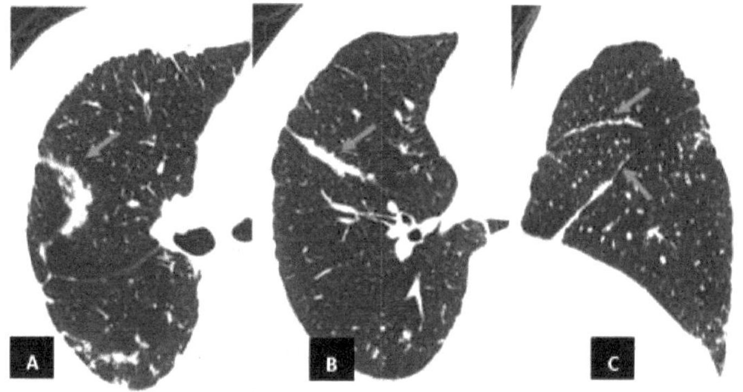

Figure 9: Juxtascissural micronodules giving a pearly appearance to the scissure.

Multiple juxtascissural micronodules (   ) confluent in places of interest to the
The small scissure (A) and the large scissure (B) give a pearly appearance to the scissures, which is best
seen in the sagittal plane (C).

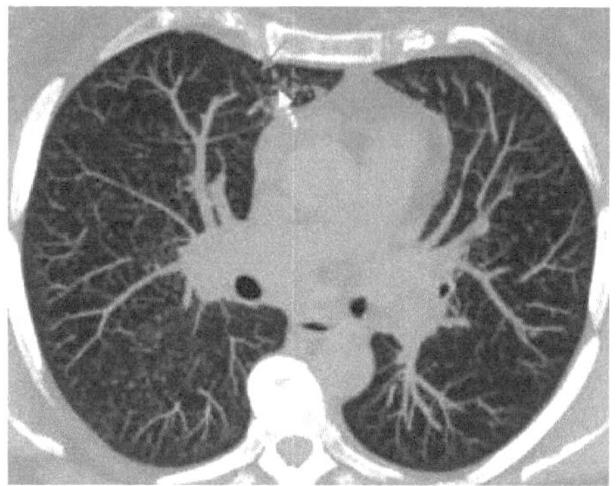

Figure 10: Subpleural pulmonary nodule in the setting of a mediastino-pulmonary sarcoidosis.

Subpleural pulmonary nodule in the ventral segment of the LSD (; surrounded by a collar of micronodules (   ) giving the characteristic appearance of

"Galaxy Sign". There are multiple micronodules of peri-lymphatic distribution in the right lung field.

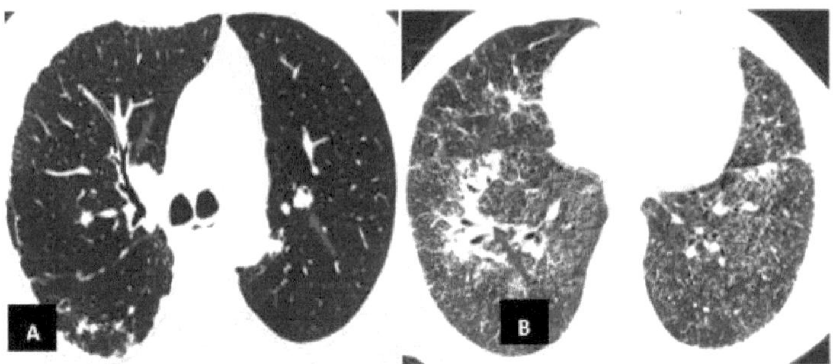

Figure 11: Peribronchovascular thickening.

Swelling around the bronchovascular structures (　) more marked in the
in the right lung of two different patients treated for mediastino-pulmonary sarcoidosis, which may be proximal perihilar (A) or more peripheral (B).

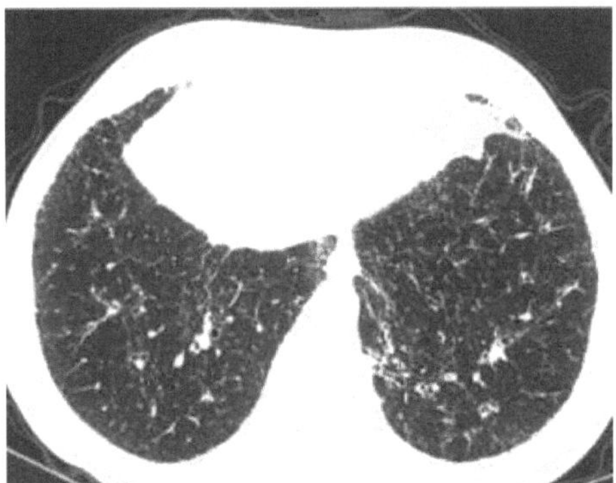

Figure 12: Bi-basal septal and non septal line thickening in mediastino-
pulmonary sarcoidosis.

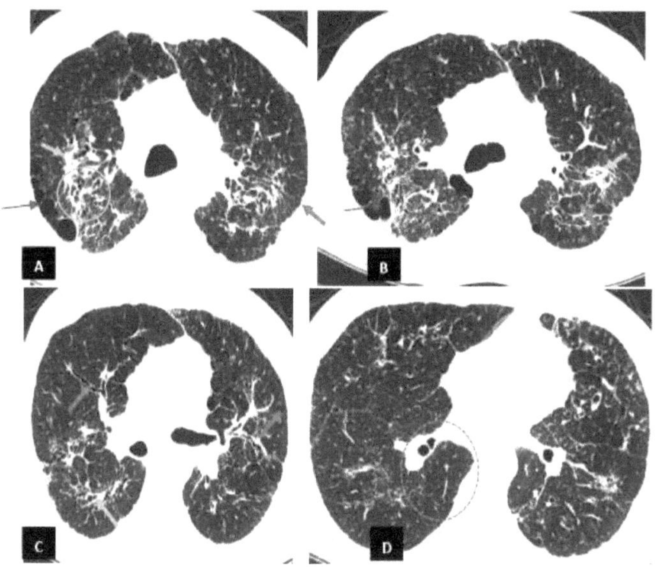

Figure 13: Mediastino-pulmonary sarcoidosis at the fibrosis stage.

Bilateral retractile fibrosis masses ( ) predominantly in the
upper regions associated with traction bronchiectasis (   ) and
significant bronchial distortion (   ). Note the focus of
associated lymphatic distribution ( ) and paracicatric   emphysema
associated (   ).

3.2.1.2 . Frequency of typical pulmonary involvement

In our series, 20 patients had predominantly nodular involvement. Typical diffuse bilateral symmetrical nodular involvement predominating in the upper and middle regions was found in 15 patients, i.e. 75% of cases.

Seven patients had fibrotic lesions in our series. Typical fibrotic lesions (traction bronchiectasis, distortion and reticulation) were predominantly diffuse or in the upper and middle regions in six patients (85.7%). (Figure 14)

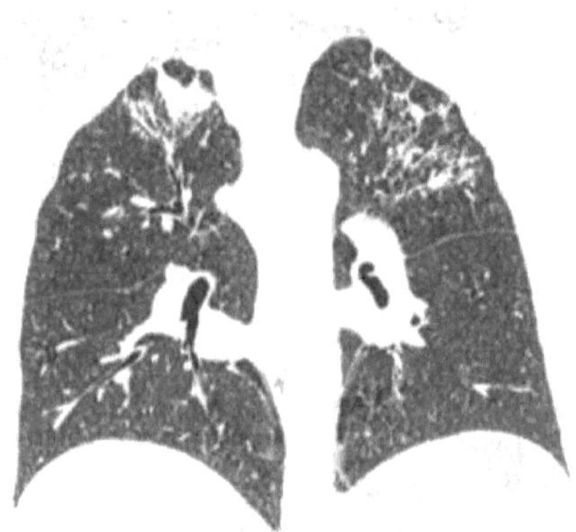

Figure 14: Mediastino-pulmonary sarcoidosis at the fibrosis stage with a predominance of elementary lesions.

3.2.1.3 Frequency of atypical lung lesions

In our series, 18 atypical conditions were found in 11 patients, i.e. 31.4% of cases. (Table III)

The most frequent atypical lesion was the atypical nodules observed in four cases:

- Nodules with ground-glass halo: N=4 (11.4%)
- Pseudotumour nodules: N=3 (8.6%). (Figure 15).

A basal predominance of elementary lesions was observed in three patients. (Figure 16).

Unilateral parenchymal involvement was found in only one case. (Figure 17)

Atelectasis and bronchial stenosis were found in three patients (8.6% of cases).

Two patients had a miliary appearance. (Figure 18).

Cavitary lesions were encountered in only one case, as well as basal honeycomb, post obstructive bronchiectasis and liquid pleural effusion.

No cases of pneumothorax were found.

Table IV: Distribution of atypical pulmonary lesions in the study population

Atypical lung disease	Number of cases	Percentage

Unilateral parenchymal disease	1	2.9
Basal predominance lesions elementary	3	8.6
Nodules with halo in frosted glass	4	11.4
Pseudotumour nodules	3	8.6
Basal honeycomb	1	2.9
Atelectasis and bronchial stenosis	3	8.6
Cavity lesions	1	2.9
Bronchiectasis post obstructive	1	2.9
Military	2	5.7
Pleural effusion	1	2.9
Pneumothorax	0	0

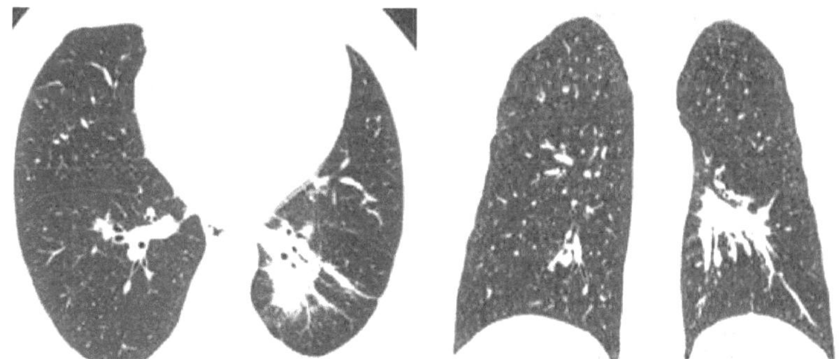

Figure 15: Sarcoidosis in its pseudotumour form

Pseudotumourous parenchymatous condensation of the LIG with a distorted aeriform bronchogram surrounded by a few micronodules of perilymphatic distribution treated with corticosteroids for 2 years. In the absence of regression of this condensation, the patient underwent a left lower lobectomy and the anatomopathological study concluded that he had pseudotumour sarcoidosis.

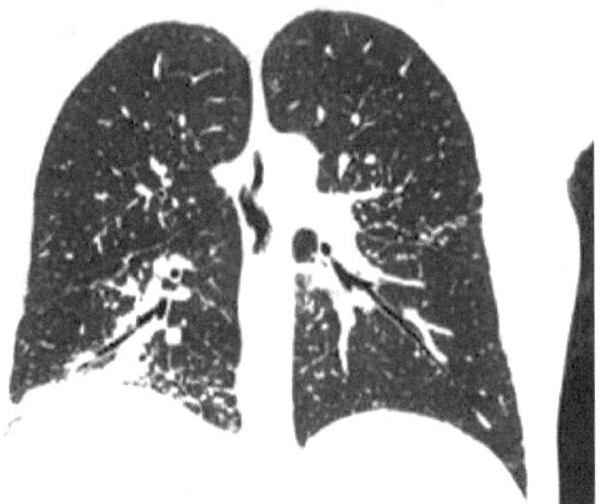

Figure 16: Atypical mediastino-pulmonary sarcoidosis with basal lesions predominating.

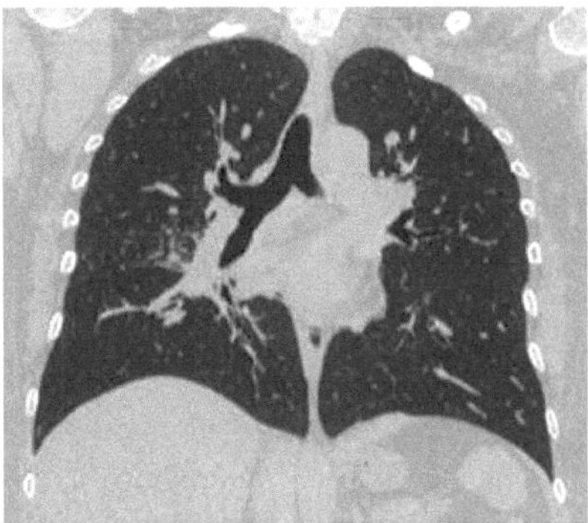

Figure 17: Atypical mediastino-pulmonary sarcoidosis with ***unilateral*** involvement.

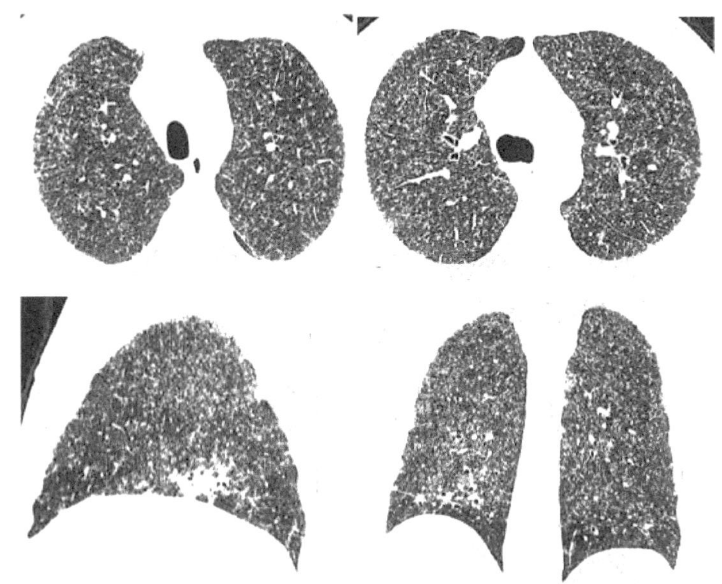

Figure 18: Atypical mediastino-pulmonary sarcoidosis in its miliary form.

Numerous ubiquitous, diffuse and bilateral micronodules associated with peribronchovascular thickening in the LID

3.2.1.4. Distribution of parenchymal lesions in the lobes

The upper and middle lobes were most affected by lesions. The right lung was more frequently affected, with the right upper lobe affected in 77.1% of N=27 patients, the right lower lobe in 51.4% of cases and the middle lobe in 74.3% of cases. (Table V)

Table V: Distribution of parenchymal lesions

in the lobes

Lobe affected	Number of patients	Percentage

Lobe touché	Nombre de patients	Pourcentage %
LSD	26	77.1
LSG	20	57.1
LM	26	74.3
LID	18	51.4
LIG	16	45.7

3.2.1.5 . Predominance of parenchymal lesions

3.2.1.5.1 Frequency of predominant parenchymal lesions

Three patients in our series had no particularly predominant elementary parenchymal lesions. In the other patients, the most frequent predominant lesions were micronodules in N=13 patients (40.6%), and nodules in N=7 patients (21.9%). Condensation was the predominant lesion in two patients. Honeycomb was the predominant lesion in only one case. (Figure 19)

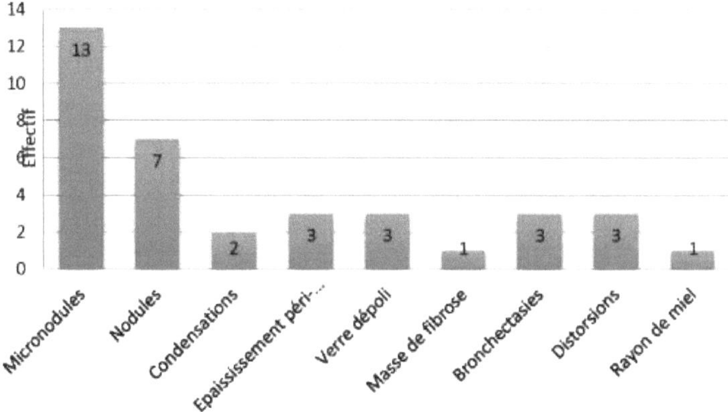

Figure 19: Distribution of predominant parenchymal lesions

in the study population

3.2.1.5.2 Topography of predominant parenchymal lesions

The locations of the predominant lesions are summarised in Table X:

The micronodules were diffusely distributed in 46.2% of cases, and more widely and/or moderately distributed in 53.8% of cases.

- The nodules were diffusely distributed in 42.9% of cases, superiorly and/or moderately distributed in 42.9% of cases, and inferiorly distributed in only one case (14.2%).

- Bronchiectasis was superior and moderate in 66.7% of cases.

- Distortions were diffuse in 66.7% of cases, and inferior in 33.3%.

Table VI: Distribution of the topography of the predominant lesions in our series

Predominant lesion	Diffuse	Superior and/or average	Lower
Micronodules (N= 13)	6 (46.2%)	7 (53.8%)	0
Nodules (N=7)	3 (42.9%)	3 (42.9%)	1 (14.2%)
Frosted glass (N=3)	1 (33.3%)	2 (66.7%)	0
Thickening bronchovascular (N=3)	1 (33.3%)	2 (66.7%)	0
Condensations (N=2)	0	1(50%)	1(50%)
Bronchiectasis (N=3)	1 (33.3%)	2 (66.7%)	0
Distortions (N=3)	2 (66.7%)	0	1 (33.3%)
Massedefibrosis (N=1)	0	1 (100%)	0
Honeycomb (N=1)	0	0	1 (100%)

3.2.2. Intra-thoracic lymph node involvement

3.2.2.1 Frequency of intra-thoracic lymph node involvement

In our series, 5 patients (14.3% of cases) had no lymph node involvement.

Hilar adenopathy was the most frequent finding in N=25 patients, i.e. 71.4% of cases. (Table VII, Figure 20).

Paratracheal adenopathy and the aorto-pulmonary window were the most frequent after hilar adenopathy. Paratracheal adenopathy was found in N=21 patients, i.e. 60% of cases, and was located on the right in the majority of patients. Adenopathies of the aorto-pulmonary window were found in N=19 patients, i.e. 54.3% of cases. (Table VII, Figure 21).

Table II: Distribution of hilar and mediastinal adenopathies in the study population

Adenopathy	Number of cases	Percentage
Hilaires	25	71.4

Paratracheal	21	60
Window aorto-pulmonary	19	54.3
Bifurcation group	12	34.3
Under carenaries	8	22.9
Mediastinal previous	14	54.3
Mediastinal posterior	5	14.3

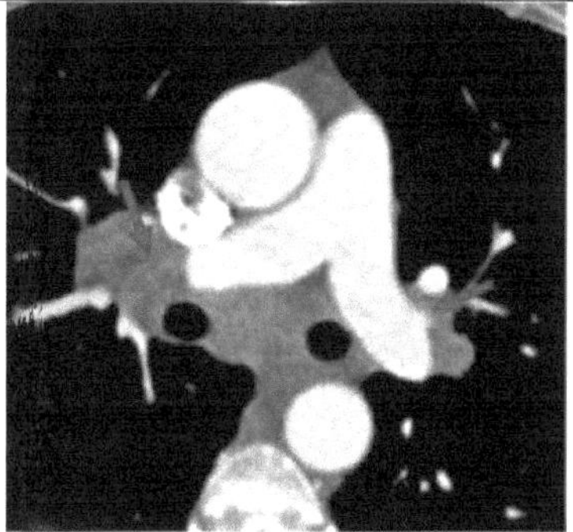

Figure 20: Bilateral, symmetrical and non-specific hilar adenomegaly.

compressive

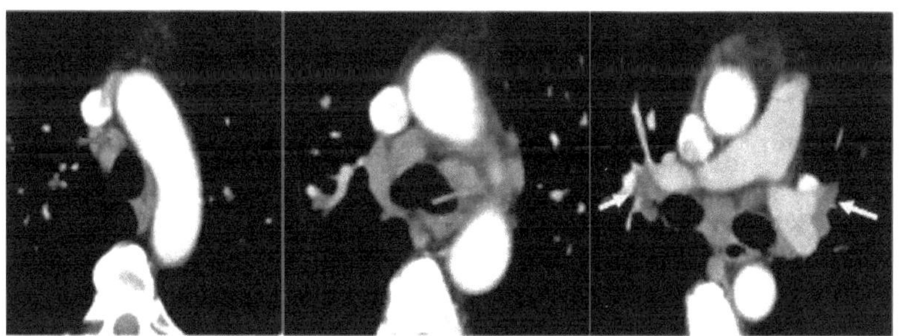

Figure 21: Common locations of mediastinal adenomegaly

Multiple mediastinal adenomegalia grouped by location involving the following chains: right lower laterotracheal (4R) () (A), aorto -   window (4R) () (B), aorto -   window (4R) () (C)

.

pulmonary (5) (   ) (B) and bilateral hilar (   ) (10).

3.2.2.2 Characteristics of atypical lymph node involvement

In our series, the atypical location of the adenopathies was
observed in five patients. These sites involved the
posterior mediastinal chain
in five patients, and the mammary chain
in a single patient.

Unilateral hilar adenopathy was seen in only two patients.

Compressive adenopathy was seen in only one patient in our series.

Calcified adenopathies were noted in two patients.

(Figure 22).

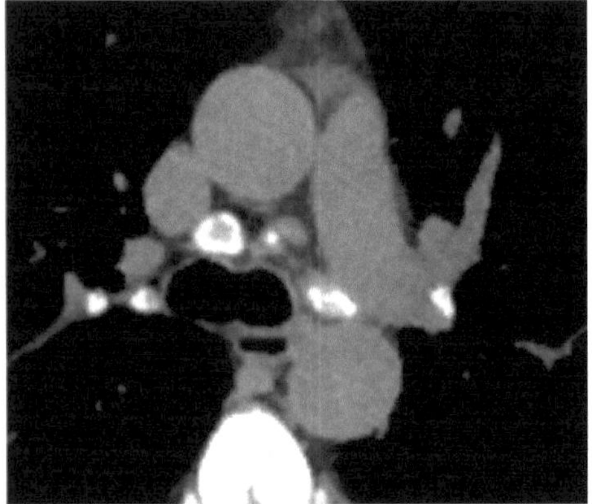

*Figure 22: "Eggshell" calcified mediastinal adenopathy Necrotic adenopathy
was seen in only one patient.*

3.2.2.3 Associated scannographic lesions

In addition to parenchymal and lymph node lesions, the CT scan
dilatation of the pulmonary artery trunk was noted in 4
cases, i.e. 11.42% of cases, and dilatation of the right cavities with signs of
pulmonary hypertension in 4 cases. (Figure 23).

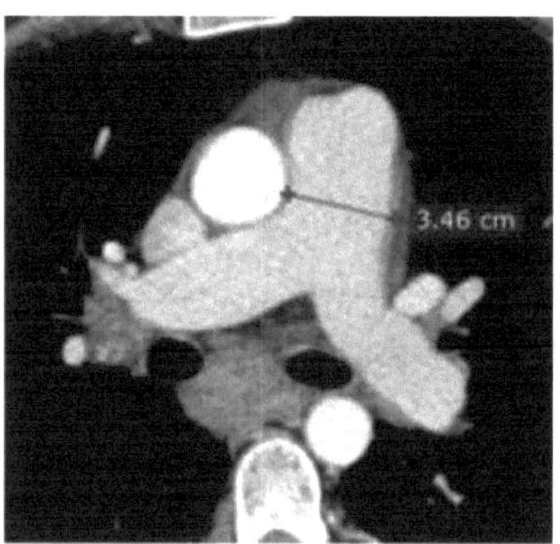

Figure 23: Dilatation of the trunk of the associated pulmonary artery

3.2.2.4 Scannographic classification of mediastinopulmonary sarcoidosis

In our series, the most frequent radiological stage was stage II, found in N=24 patients (68.6%), followed by stage IV, found in N=5 patients (14.3%). Stages I and III were equally less frequent (8.6% of cases). (Figure 24).

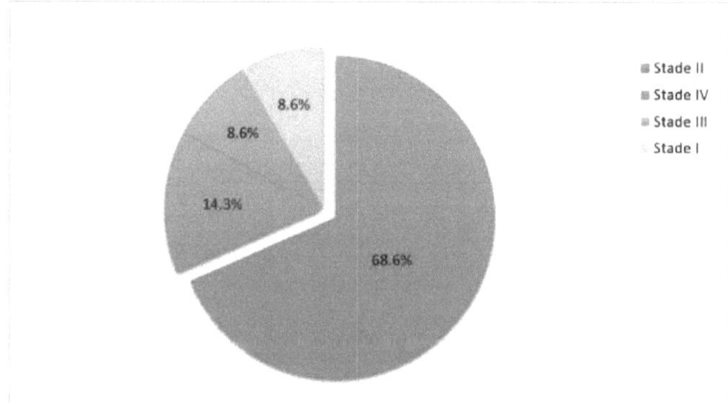

Figure 24: Distribution of sarcoidosis scan stages in the study population

CHAPTER 3

D) <u>Discussion</u>

Radiological diagnosis

Bilateral symmetrical hilar lymphadenopathy is a feature of sarcoidosis and may help to distinguish sarcoidosis from other conditions responsible for hilar and mediastinal lymphadenopathy.

The typical radiographic manifestation of parenchymal lung involvement by sarcoidosis is diffuse micronodules predominating in the upper and middle parts of the lungs (14).

On chest CT, peri lymphatic micronodules are the most common abnormality in pulmonary sarcoidosis (178). In the absence of parenchymal involvement, bilateral hilar lymphadenopathy is present in 98% of cases (20).

1) Standard chest X-ray

Chest radiography is still a fundamental tool in the diagnosis of sarcoidosis (11). Chest radiographic abnormalities are seen in over 90% of patients with thoracic sarcoidosis (12). Based on the appearance of the chest X-ray, the disease is divided into five radiological stages described by Siltzbach (13), ranging from no visible abnormality (stage 0) to terminal fibrosis. This classification of sarcoidosis is based on the presence of hilar or mediastinal adenopathies, and also the presence of pulmonary infiltration without or with fibrosis (14).

This classification is justified by its diagnostic and prognostic value, and the likelihood of spontaneous resolution, which generally decreases as the disease progresses (15). However, it has been shown that chest radiography is not a reliable indicator of lung function (15).

Radiological stages I and II are the most frequent according to several authors. (Table IX)

In our study population, the most frequent radiological stage was stage III, found in 34.4% of cases, followed by stage II, found in 25.7% of cases.

Table IX: Radiographic classification of sarcoidosis in the literature and in our series.

literature and in our series.

Study	Country	Year	Stadium				
			Stage 0	Stage I	II	Stage III	Stage IV
Tavana et al. (16)	Nigeria	2015	-	69%	10.9%	14.5%	5.5%
Nunes et al (17)	France	2005	8-16%	25 65%	14-49%	9.8%	5.4%
Bart et al. (18)	Switzerland	2005	5-10%	50%	25%	15%	5-10%
Morar and Feldman(19)	South Africa	2022	2.9%	23.5%	48%	15.7%	9.8%
Sreeja et al (20)	India	2022	-	40 50%	30-40%	15 20%	2-5%
Our Series	Tunisia	2023	11.4%	17.1%	25.7%	34.3%	11.4%

2) Data from thoracic CT scan

Thoracic CT provides a more thorough and sensitive investigation for the detection of parenchymal abnormalities and thoracic adenopathies (21). It is also useful when there is a strong clinical suspicion of complications such as aspergilloma, concomitant infection or malignancy (22).

Computed tomography of the chest shows lymphadenopathy and pulmonary infiltration with better accuracy than X-rays (11).

In our study, parenchymal involvement with elementary lesions occurred in 32 patients, i.e. 91.4% of cases. Lymph node involvement occurred in 30 patients (85.7% of cases), which is in line with the results of the literature (23), as shown in Table X below.

Table X: Frequency of parenchymal and lymph node involvement
in the literature and in our series.

Study	Country	Year	Damage	Damage

			parenchymal	lymph node
Fourati (23)	Tunisia	2009	93%	100%
Muller et al. (24)	Canada	1989	80%	80%
Desloques (25)	France	2018	85%	85%
Our study	Tunisia	2023	91.4%	85.7%

2.1. Parenchymal involvement

2.1.1 Characteristics of elementary parenchymal lesions

A) The typical radiographic manifestation of lung parenchymal involvement by sarcoidosis consists of diffuse peri lymphatic micronodules predominating in the upper and middle parts of the lungs (15,26). These micronodules, visible on CT scan, are formed by the fusion of microscopic sarcoid granulomas (15), and may fuse into irregular nodules surrounded by micronodules (galaxy sign) (27). Micronodules were the most frequent type of involvement in our study, found in 71.4% of cases, which is consistent with the results of the literature where they exist in 75% and 85.2% of patients respectively in Muller et al. (15) and Fourati (23). (Table X)

B) Nodules are rounded pulmonary opacities predominating in the peripheral and parahilar regions and measuring up to 3 cm in diameter (15). A lesion larger than 3 cm is a mass (28). Parenchymal involvement is generally present in 25% of cases (29,24).

C) Peribronchovascular thickening results from the presence of an aggregate of granulomas in the lymphatic system of the peribronchovascular connective sheaths (23). It is a regular or irregular thickening of the bronchial walls and vascular contours.

- Nodular lesions (micronodules and nodules) and peribronchovascular thickening are the two most frequent elementary lesions in our series, and this is consistent with the results of the literature, as illustrated in the table.

- Nodular lesions were frequent in our series, which is explained by the frequency of atypical nodules and the frequency of stage II lesions.

D) Condensations result from the confluence of nodular lesions, and predominate in the upper and middle regions of the lungs (15). Their frequency in our series was 20%, which is consistent with the literature.

E) Ground-glass opacities are the main radiological lesion in rare cases (30). They may be due to alveolitis or developing pulmonary fibrosis, and generally occur in 21-31% of cases (31), which is consistent with the results of our study. In Fourati's study, they occurred in 51.8% of cases, given the high frequency of the

fibrosis.

F) Septal thickening results from an agglomeration of granulomas in the lymphatics of the interlobular septa, so the typical distribution suggestive of sarcoidosis is perilymphatic (15).

In our series, this radiological sign was present in 43.3% of cases.

G) Cavitary lesions are present in less than 5% of cases at initial presentation, and accompany a very active disease. Most of the apparent cavities seen on CT images are in fact bullae or cysts that have developed in the advanced fibrocystic stage of sarcoidosis (32). These cavities are lined with dense fibrous tissue and not granulomas, as cavitation most commonly occurs in areas of advanced fibrosis (33). The thickening of the cavity walls is reduced under treatment. The risk is that of infection, particularly aspergillosis grafting with haemoptysis (27).

In our series, the cavitary lesion was found in only one patient.

H) Fibrosis lesions include broncovascular and scissural distortions, traction bronchiectasis, honeycomb, intralobular reticulations and fibrosis masses.

The distortions are mainly of upper and middle topography in the lung, mainly affecting the bronchus of the dorsal segment of the right upper lobe (33). Bronchial distortions with or without a fibrosis mass are associated with TVO

(27). The honeycomb is associated with a frank restrictive syndrome and a marked reduction in DLCO; this lesion is most often apical or in the middle peri-hilar stage (27).

Fibrosis masses form during long-term evolution and are usually located at the apex.

In our series, these lesions were present in 20% of cases, and this is consistent with the literature, as shown in Table XI below.

Table III: Frequency of elementary lesions in the literature and in our series.

Elementary lesions	Fourati (23) Tunisia 2009	Muller et al. (24)	Our study
Micronodules	85.2%	75%	71.4%
Nodules	59.2%	25%	51.4%
Condensations parenchymal	25.9%	-	20%
Frosted glass	51.8%	-	28.6%
Crazy paving	3.7%	-	5.7%
Thickening bronchovascular	70.4%	60%	40%
Septal lines	66.7%	50%	34.3%
Bronchiectasis of traction	33.3%	-	20%
Scissural distortion	48.1%	-	20%
Distortion bronchovascular	48.1%	-	20%
Intra joints lobular	18.5%	-	14.3%
Honeycomb	18.5%	-	8.6%
Fibrosis mass	11.1%	20%	8.6%

Cavities	3.7%	-	2.9%
Aspergilloma	-	-	0
Signs of PH	0	-	8,6%

A.1.2. Manifestations of typical parenchymal involvement :

Parenchymal involvement is typical when it has the following characteristics (29):

A) Nodular lesions (micronodules and nodules)

Perilymphatically diffused micronodules are the most common typical involvement in sarcoidosis. Computed tomography shows small (2 to 4 mm in diameter), well-limited, bilateral, symmetrical, rounded lesions predominating in the upper and middle regions of the lung in (75 to 90%) of cases. These micronodules coalesce into larger nodules (>5mm).

B) Lymphatic diffusion of lesions :

It diffuses into the peribronchovascular interstitium, the subpleural interstitium and the interlobular septa.

In our series, 20 patients had predominant nodular involvement. Typical diffuse bilateral symmetrical nodular involvement predominating in the upper and middle regions was found in 15 patients, i.e. 75% of cases, and this is consistent with the results of the literature (29).

C) Fibrotic changes :

Typical fibrosis lesions include reticulations, architectural distortion and traction bronchiectasis (29), with an upper and middle predominance of these lesions.

Seven patients had fibrotic lesions in our series. Typical fibrotic lesions (traction bronchiectasis, distortion and reticulation) were predominantly diffuse or in the upper and middle regions in six patients (85.7%).

D) Elementary parenchymal abnormalities predominate in the upper and middle zones.

A.1.3. Manifestations of atypical lung disease :

Atypical involvement is rarely seen in mediastino-pulmonary sarcoidosis. They pose problems of differential diagnosis, and are usually found in elderly subjects

(23,33).

In our series, 11 patients or 31.4% of cases had atypical lesions, and this is somewhat similar to the results of the Maulat study where these lesions existed in 21.7% of cases. The differences in the frequency of atypical parenchymal lesions with the literature are due to the small number of patients in our series and also to the higher frequency of elderly subjects in our series.

A) Atypical nodules

They point to another pathology. They occur in 17% of cases in Fourati's study of 29 cases (23). In our series, four patients (11.4% of cases) had atypical nodules.

- Pseudotumour nodules :

These are nodules with lymphatic distribution or solitary nodules. They pose the problem of differential diagnosis with secondary lesions and lymphomas (23). In our series, these nodules were present in three patients, i.e. 8.6% of cases, which is consistent with the literature.

- Nodules with ground glass halo :

They pose the problem of differential diagnosis with patients having opportunistic pulmonary infections in immunocompromised patients (aspergillosis), and kaposi sarcoma. In our series, these nodules occurred in 11.4% of cases.

B) Unilateral parenchymal involvement :

Atypical involvement is seen when the parenchymal involvement is unilateral (35), and this poses the problem of differential diagnosis with carcinomatous lymphangitis (23). Only one patient in our series had strictly unilateral involvement, which is consistent with the literature.

C) Basal predominance of parenchymal lesions :

The elementary parenchymal lesions of sarcoidosis rarely predominate in the basal regions of the lung.

In our series, three patients had a predominance of elementary lesions in the basal regions.

8) Frosted glass hyperdensities :

They were found in 28% of cases in our series.

D) The basal honeycomb :

The honeycomb is most often apical or in the middle perihilar layer, unlike in idiopathic pulmonary fibrosis where it is peripheral basal and subpleural(30). Only one patient in our series had basal honeycomb.

E) Atelectasis and bronchial stenosis :

Obstruction of the lobar or segmental bronchi by small endobronchial granulomas or enlarged peribronchial lymph nodes leads to atelectasis (36).

In our series, three patients (8.6%) had atelectasis, which is consistent with the literature.

F) Cavities :

In our series, cavities were present in only one case, and this is consistent with the literature.

G) Post-obstructive bronchiectasis :

These are post-obstructive bronchial dilations in the non-fibrosing stages of the disease, related to the endobronchial development of large granulomas early in the disease (23).

In our series, only one patient had post obstructive bronchiectasis.

H) Militaries:

These lesions are very rare (<1%) in cases. Their presence poses the problem of differential diagnosis with tuberculosis, secondary lesions and pneumoconiosis (37).

In our series, two patients presented with miliary disease.

I) Pleural involvement :

Pleural involvement is very rare in sarcoidosis, occurring in only 1 to 4% of cases. Pleural effusion is generally small and disappears within two to three months (38). Pneumothorax results from rupture of an emphysematous bulla in the late fibrotic stages of the disease (38).

In our series, pleural effusion was present in only one patient. Pneumothorax was not present in any case.

The following table (XII) shows the frequency of atypical parenchymal involvement in the literature and in our series.

Table IV: Comparison of the frequency of lung damage atypical between our study and the study by Fourati (23)

Atypical disease	Fourati (23) Tunisia 2009	Our series
Nodulespseudo tumor	17%	8.6%
Nodules with halo in frosted glass	0	11.4%
Unilateral damage	0	2.9%
Basal predominance lesions	0	8.6%
Basal honeycomb	10%	2.9%
Atelectasisand bronchial stenosis	5%	8.6%
Bronchiectasis post obstructive	10%	2.9%
miliary	0	5.7%

Cavities	3.4%	2.9%
Pleural effusion	3.4%	2.9%
Pneumothorax	0	0

A.1.4. Distribution of parenchymal lesions in the lobes

Involvement of the upper and middle lobes was the most frequent. The right lung was more frequently affected in the study by Adila et al (39) and the study by Fourati (23), and this is consistent with the results of our series (Table XIII).

Table V:Distribution of parenchymal lesions in the lobes

in the literature and in our study.

Lobe affected	Adila et al (39)	Fourati (23)	Our series
Lobe touché	Adila et al. (39)	Fourati (23)	Notre série
LSD	80.8%	70.6%	77.1%
LSG	71.8%	58.8%	57.1%
LM	80.8%	85.3%	74.3%
LID	-	58.8%	51.4%
LIG	-	41.2%	45.7%

A.1.5. Predominance of parenchymal lesions

A.1.5.1.   Frequency of predominant parenchymal lesions

Nodular lesions and peribronchovascular thickening were the most frequent predominant lesions in the literature (23,40), and this is consistent with the results of our study. Table

Condensation was the predominant lesion in 6% of cases in Augier et al, and this is consistent with the results of our study.

Bronchiectasis and distortion were the most frequent predominant fibrosis lesions in Fourati's study (23), and this is consistent with the results of our study.

(Table XIV)

***Table VI: Frequency of predominant lesions and comparison
with literature results.***

Predominant lesion	Fourati (23)	Augier et al. (41)	Our study
Micronodules	27.9%	27%	43.8% (N=13)
Condensations	-	6%	6.25%
Nodules	18.5%	7%	21.9%
Peripheral thickening bronchovascular	14.8%	12%	9.4%
Frosted glass	14.8%	11%	9.4%
Fibrosis mass	3.7%	9%	3.1%
Bronchiectasis	7.4%	-	9.4%
Distortions	11.1%	-	9.4%
Honeycomb	3.7%	-	3.1%

A.1.5.2. Topography of predominant parenchymal lesions

In our series, we noted a preferential distribution of lesions in the upper and/or middle regions or in a diffuse fashion. This is consistent with the pathogenesis of sarcoidosis, which, due to lymphatic tropism, is preferentially located in the posterior and upper regions, especially on the right, where lymphatic drainage is most impaired.

A.2. Intra-thoracic lymph node disease

A.2.1. Frequency of intra-thoracic lymph node involvement

The presence of bilateral, symmetrical hilar and mediastinal adenopathies, satellite to the tracheobronchial axis, voluminous and non-compressive, is typical of lymph node involvement in sarcoidosis (35).

In our series, the lymph nodes most frequently involved were the hilar nodes (71.4%) and the paratracheal nodes (60%). This is consistent with the results of the literature. (Table XV)

-       The aorto-pulmonary window was affected in 54.3% of cases, which is consistent with the results of our study.

-       The anterior mediastinal chain was involved in 54.3% of cases, in agreement with the results of Fourati (23).

-       The subcarinal chain was affected in 42.85% of cases. The bifurcation group was affected in 34.3% of cases. These differences in frequency can be explained by the small number of patients in our series.

Table VII: Distribution of intrathoracic lymph node involvement in our study and in the literature.

Damage lymph node	Desloques (131)	Fourati(13 5)	Our series
Hilaires	97%	86.2%	71.4%
Paratracheal	71%	86.2%	60%
Aorto pulmonary	76%	69%	54.3%
Group bifurcation	-	79.3%	34.3%
Under carenaries	21%	79.3%	22.9%
Mediastinal previous	16%	51.7%	54.3%
Mediastinal posterior	-	20.7%	14.3%

A.2.2. Characteristics of atypical lymph node involvement

A) Mediastinal adenopathy in atypical locations

These locations involve the diaphragmatic or cardiophrenic lymph nodes, the internal mammary chain and the posterior mediastinal chain. In the study by Fourati, an atypical location of mediastinal adenopathies was found in 24% of cases, and this is consistent with the results of our series where they existed in 18% of patients. Involvement of the posterior mediastinal chain was noted in five patients, and involvement of the internal mammary chain was noted in only one patient.

B) Unilateral and/or asymmetric hilar adenopathy

Bilateral and symmetric hilar lymphadenopathy is atypical of sarcoidosis (42). Unilateral and asymmetric hilar lymphadenopathy is rare, occurring in less than 5% of cases. It is more common in subjects aged over 50 (43).

This condition poses the problem of differential diagnosis with tuberculosis, lymphoma and secondary lesions (44).

In our series, unilateral hilar adenopathy was seen in two patients (5.7% of cases), which is consistent with the literature.

C) Calcified nature of adenopathies (eggshell calcifications)

They suggest silicosis, pneumoconiosis and amyloidosis (42). Sarcoidosis is the most common cause of this form of adenopathy calcification in patients without occupational exposure to silicosis or pneumoconiosis (34).

Calcified lymph nodes increase in frequency with the age of the disease, occurring in 3% of cases after 5 years and in 20% of cases after 10 years (34).

In our series, calcified adenopathies were noted in two patients.

D) Necrotic adenopathy

These are hypodense adenopathies with necrotic centres. They are an exceptional presentation in sarcoidosis according to the study by Maulat (45). Maulat believes that their frequency is underestimated because contrast is not routinely injected.

In our series, the atypical location of adenopathies was observed in five patients.

These involved the posterior mediastinal chain in five patients, and the internal mammary chain in one patient.

E) Compressive nature of adenopathy

Adenopathies in sarcoidosis do not generally compress adjacent structures (vessels and airways) (42).

In our series, the compressive nature was noted in only one case, where a patient had large hilar adenopathies compressing the pulmonary artery.

A.3. Associated scannographic lesions

Radiological signs of pulmonary hypertension and dilatation of right cavities may be observed. In pulmonary hypertension, signs of distortion, fibrosis and compression of the pulmonary artery by lymph nodes may suggest sarcoidosis as a cause (45). Mycetomas may also be observed in very advanced forms of sarcoidosis. They may be the site of an aspergillary infection (10).

In our series, CT scans revealed dilatation of the pulmonary artery trunk in 4 cases, i.e. 11.42% of cases, and dilatation of the right cavities with signs of pulmonary hypertension in 4 cases.

Mycetomas were not noted in any cases.

CHAPTER 4

E) <u>Conclusion</u>

The clinical presentation of sarcoidosis depends on the intensity and duration of the inflammation and the organs involved. The phenotypes of the disease are highly variable, ranging from completely asymptomatic forms with pulmonary alterations found incidentally on routine chest X-rays to sub-acute and acute clinical presentations. Chest X-ray abnormalities are observed in more than 90% of patients with thoracic sarcoidosis, both in the literature and in our series (12).

Thoracic computed tomography plays a very important role in the diagnosis and monitoring of the disease. It provides a more thorough and sensitive study for the detection of parenchymal abnormalities and thoracic adenopathies. Micronodules were the most frequent lesion in our study, found in 71.4% of cases, which is consistent with the results of the literature. (23,24)

References

1. Hillerdal G, Nöu E, Osterman K, Schmekel B. Sarcoidosis: epidemiology and prognosis. A 15-year European study. Am Rev Respir Dis. 1984 Jul;130(1):29-32.

2. Baughman RP, Teirstein AS, Judson MA, Rossman MD, Yeager H, Bresnitz EA, et al. Clinical characteristics of patients in a case control study of sarcoidosis. Am J Respir Crit Care Med. 2001 Nov 15;164(10 Pt 1):1885-9.

3. Spagnolo P, Rossi G, Trisolini R, Sverzellati N, Baughman RP, Wells AU. Pulmonary sarcoidosis. The Lancet Respiratory Medicine. 2018 May;6(5):389-402.

4. Baughman RP, Iannuzzi MC. Diagnosis of sarcoidosis: when is a peek good enough? Chest. 2000 Apr;117(4):931-2.

5. Lemerre D, Caron F, Delval O, Jm G, Hira M, Jc M, et al. Thyroid manifestations in sarcoidosis: a case report. Revue De Pneumologie Clinique [Internet]. 2008 Feb 22 [cited 2023 Jul 27]

6. Valeyre D, Brauner M, Bernaudin JF, Carbonnelle E, Duchemann B, Rotenberg C, et al. Differential diagnosis of pulmonary sarcoidosis: a review. Front Med. 2023 May 12; 10:1150751.

7. BART PA, ZUBER JP, LEIMGRUBER A, SPERTINI F. Sarcoidosis: new pathogenic and therapeutic concepts for an "old" disease: Allergo-immunology. Rev méd suisse. 2005 ;1(15):1026-38.

8. Mahler DA, Wells CK. Evaluation of clinical methods for rating dyspnea. Chest. 1988 Mar ;93(3):580-6.

9. Baughman RP, Culver DA, Judson MA. A Concise Review of Pulmonary Sarcoidosis. Am J Respir Crit Care Med. 2011 Mar 1;183(5):573-81.

10. Criado E, Sánchez M, Ramírez J, Arguis P, de Caralt TM, Perea RJ, et al. Pulmonary sarcoidosis: typical and atypical manifestations at highresolution CT with pathologic correlation. Radiographics. 2010 Oct;30(6):1567-86.

11. Lynch JP, Kazerooni EA, Gay SE. Pulmonary sarcoidosis. Clin Chest Med. 1997 Dec;18(4):755-85.

12. Baughman RP, Teirstein AS, Judson MA, Rossman MD, Yeager H, Bresnitz EA, et al. Clinical characteristics of patients in a case control study of sarcoidosis. Am J Respir Crit Care Med. 2001 Nov 15;164(10 Pt 1):1885-9.

13. Siltzbach LE, James DG, Neville E, Turiaf J, Battesti JP, Sharma OP, et al. Course and prognosis of sarcoidosis around the world. Am J Med. 1974 Dec;57(6):847-52.

14. Statement on sarcoidosis. Joint Statement of the American Thoracic Society (ATS), the European Respiratory Society (ERS) and the World Association of Sarcoidosis and Other Granulomatous Disorders (WASOG)

15. Lee GM, Pope K, Meek L, Chung JH, Hobbs SB, Walker CM. Sarcoidosis: A Diagnosis of Exclusion. American Journal of Roentgenology. 2020 Jan;214(1):50-8.

16. Tavana S, Alizadeh M, Mohajerani SA, Hashemian SM. Pulmonary and extra-pulmonary manifestations of sarcoidosis. Niger Med J. 2015;56(4):258-62.

17. Nunes H, Soler P, Valeyre D. Pulmonary sarcoidosis. Allergy. 2005 May;60(5):565-82.

18. BART PA, ZUBER JP, LEIMGRUBER A, SPERTINI F. Sarcoidosis: new pathogenic and therapeutic concepts for an "old" disease: Allergo-immunology. Rev méd suisse. 2005 ;1(15):1026-38.

19. Morar R, Feldman C. Sarcoidosis in Johannesburg, South Africa: A retrospective study. Afr J Thoracic Crit Care Med. 2022 Dec 19 ;150-6.

20. Sreeja C, Priyadarshini A, Premika, Nachiammai N. Sarcoidosis - A review article. J Oral Maxillofac Pathol. 2022;26(2):242.

21. Desloques L. Imaging of extrathoracic thoracic manifestations of sarcoidosis. Congress presented at; 2018; Imagerie Polyclinique Cote Basque Sud - Saint Jean de Luz.

22. Nunes H, Brillet PY, Valeyre D, Brauner MW, Wells AU. Imaging in sarcoidosis. Semin Respir Crit Care Med. 2007 Feb;28(1):102-20.

23. Fourati H. Imagery of sarcoidosis: Retrospective study of 29 cases of mediastino-pulmonary sarcoidosis, and iconographic review of its extra-thoracic manifestations [Thesis]. Faculté de médecine de sfax; 2009.

24. Muller N, Kullnig P, Miller R. The CT findings of pulmonary sarcoidosis: analysis of 25 patients. American Journal of Roentgenology. 1989 Jun;152(6):1179-82.

25. Desloques L. Imaging of extrathoracic thoracic manifestations of sarcoidosis. Congress presented at; 2018; Imagerie Polyclinique Cote Basque Sud - Saint Jean de Luz.

26. Bein ME, Putman CE, McLoud TC, Mink JH. A reevaluation of intrathoracic lymphadenopathy in sarcoidosis. AJR Am J Roentgenol. 1978 Sep;131(3):409-15.

27. Uzunhan Y, Jeny F, Crockett F, Piver D, Kambouchner M, Valeyre D, et al. Pulmonary sarcoidosis: clinical aspects and treatment modalities. La Revue de Médecine Interne. 2016 Sep 1;37(9):594- 607.

28. Hansell DM, Bankier AA, MacMahon H, McLoud TC, Müller NL, Remy J. Fleischner Society: glossary of terms for thoracic imaging. Radiology. 2008 Mar;246(3):697-722.

29. Criado E, Sánchez M, Ramírez J, Arguis P, de Caralt TM, Perea RJ, et al. Pulmonary sarcoidosis: typical and atypical manifestations at highresolution CT with pathologic correlation. Radiographics. 2010 Oct;30(6):1567-86.

30. Uzunhan Y, Jeny F, Crockett F, Piver D, Kambouchner M, Valeyre D, et al. Pulmonary sarcoidosis: clinical aspects and modalities. therapeutics. The Journal of Internal Medicine. 2016 Sep 1;37(9):594- 607.

31. Augier A, Brillet PY, Duperon F, Nunes H, Valeyre D, Brauner M. CT analysis of 500 cases of pulmonary sarcoidosis. Journal de Radiologie. 2005 Oct 1;86(10):1385.

32. Ichikawa Y, Fujimoto K, Shiraishi T, Oizumi K. Primary cavitary sarcoidosis: high-resolution CT findings. AJR Am J Roentgenol. 1994 Sep;163(3):745.

33. Maulat I. CT aspects of rare and/or atypical forms of sarcoidosis. [Thèse de doctorat en médecine]. [Paris]; 2003.

34. Chiles C. Imaging features of thoracic sarcoidosis. Semin Roentgenol. 2002 Jan;37(1):82-93.

35. Javot L, Tala S, Scala-Bertola J, Massy N, Trenque T, Baldin B, et al. Sarcoidosis and anti-TNF: a paradoxical class effect? Analysis of cases in the French Pharmacovigilance database and review of the literature. Therapies. 2011 Mar 1;66(2):149-54.

36. Lenique F, Brauner MW, Grenier P, Battesti JP, Loiseau A, Valeyre D. CT assessment of bronchi in sarcoidosis: endoscopic and pathologic correlations. Radiology. 1995 Feb;194(2):419-23.

37. Wells A. High resolution computed tomography in sarcoidosis: a clinical perspective. Sarcoidosis Vasc Diffuse Lung Dis. 1998 Sep;15(2):140-6.

38. Soskel NT, Sharma OP. Pleural involvement in sarcoidosis. Curr Opin Pulm Med. 2000 Sep;6(5):455-68.

39. Adila F, Boucetta R, Chiba F, Brahimi T, Ziane F, Zitouni A. Thoracic imaging of sarcoidosis. Revue des Maladies Respiratoires Actualités. 2022 Jan 1;14(1):219.

40. CT analysis of 500 cases of pulmonary sarcoidosis. Journal of Radiology. 2005 Oct 1;86(10):1385.

41. Augier A, Brillet PY, Duperon F, Nunes H, Valeyre D, Brauner M. CT analysis of 500 cases of pulmonary sarcoidosis. Journal de Radiologie. 2005 Oct 1;86(10):1385.

42. Valeyre D, Brauner M, Bernaudin JF, Carbonnelle E, Duchemann B, Rotenberg C, et al. Differential diagnosis of pulmonary sarcoidosis: a review. Front Med. 2023 May 12; 10:1150751.

43. Park HJ, Jung JI, Chung MH, Song SW, Kim HL, Baik JH, et al. Typical and atypical manifestations of intrathoracic sarcoidosis. Korean J Radiol. 2009;10(6):623-31.

44. Rockoff S, Rohatgi P. Unusual manifestations of thoracic sarcoidosis. American Journal of Roentgenology. 1985 Mar;144(3):513-28.

45. Maulat I. CT aspects of rare and/or atypical forms of sarcoidosis. [Thèse de

doctorat en médecine]. [Paris];
2003.

46. Nunes H, Humbert M, Capron F, Brauner M, Sitbon O, Battesti JP, et al. Pulmonary hypertension associated with sarcoidosis: mechanisms, haemodynamics and prognosis. Thorax. 2006 Jan;61(1):68-74.

Appendix 1: Classification of dyspnoea according to the modified mMRC dyspnoea scale.

Stadium	Description
0	No dyspnoea, except in cases of severe physical exertion.
1	Dyspnoea when walking quickly on the flat or on a gentle slope.
2	Dyspnoea when walking on level ground following someone your own age or having to stop to catch your breath when walking on level ground at your own pace.
3	Dyspnoea requiring you to stop and catch your breath after a few minutes or a hundred metres on flat ground.
4	Dyspnoea making it impossible to leave the house, dyspnoea when dressing or undressing.

Appendix 2: Radiological stages of sarcoidosis according to the Siltzbach classification.

Stadium Radiological	Description
I	Telar mediastinal adenopathy (often bilateral) without pulmonary infiltrates
II	Association of mediastinal and hilar adenopathies (often bilateral) with pulmonary infiltrates
III	Lung infiltrates without adenopathy
IV	Pulmonary fibrosis

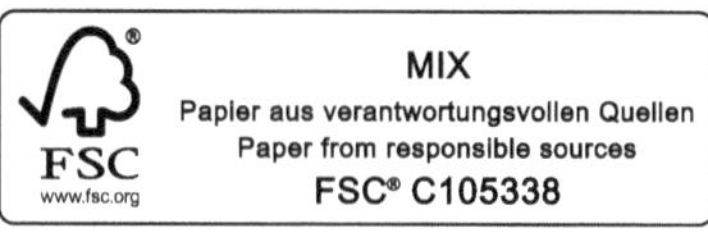

Printed by Books on Demand GmbH, Norderstedt / Germany